OSCAR OCEAN AND THE BIG STRETCH

Written by Josephine NC Groenhart
Illustrated by Eloise Biernat

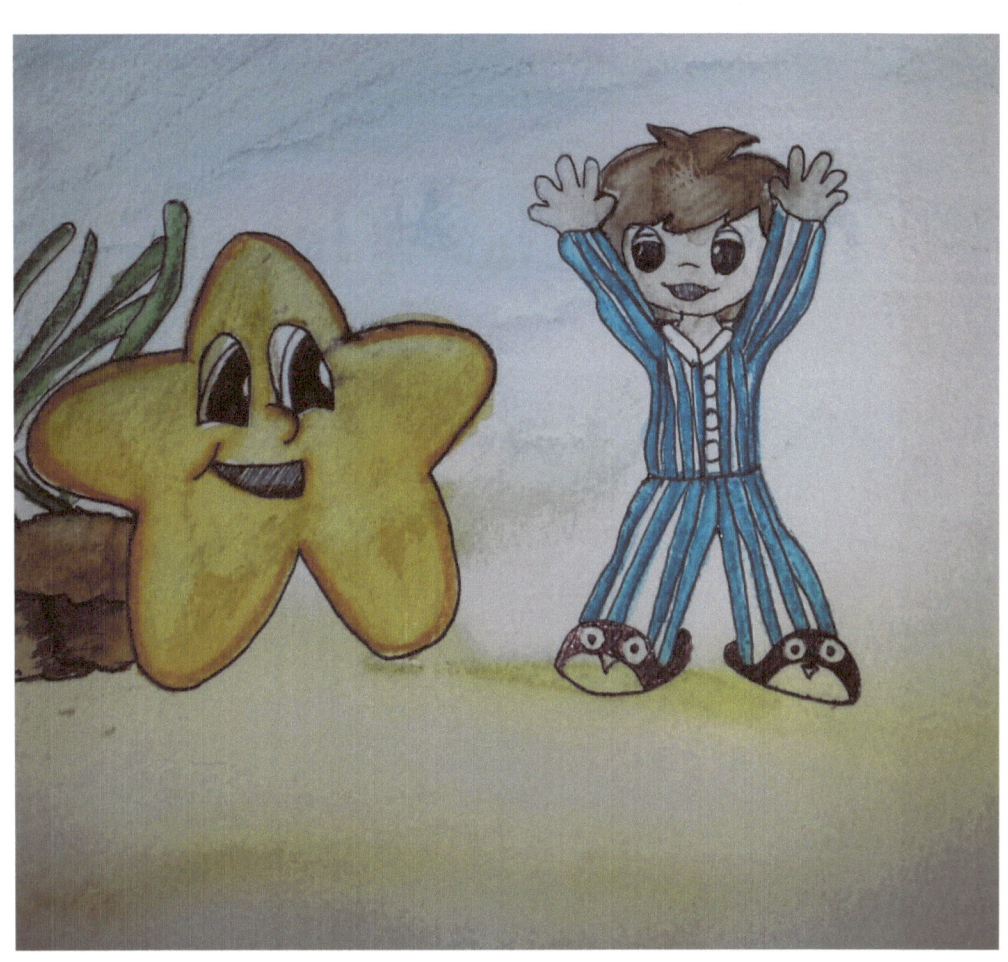

DEDICATION

For Isaac and Oakley. My two cheeky monkeys!

ACKNOWLEDGMENTS

With special thanks to Eloise for her amazing illustrations, Ed for all your encouragement and Isaac, Oakley and all the children in our centre who have helped me put this together for you all.

THANK YOU

Dimming down the light mum said "Good night,"
Oscar rolled over and snuggled-in tight.
Sammy Seahorse looked up at him and said,
"Oscar you need to stretch before you go to
bed."

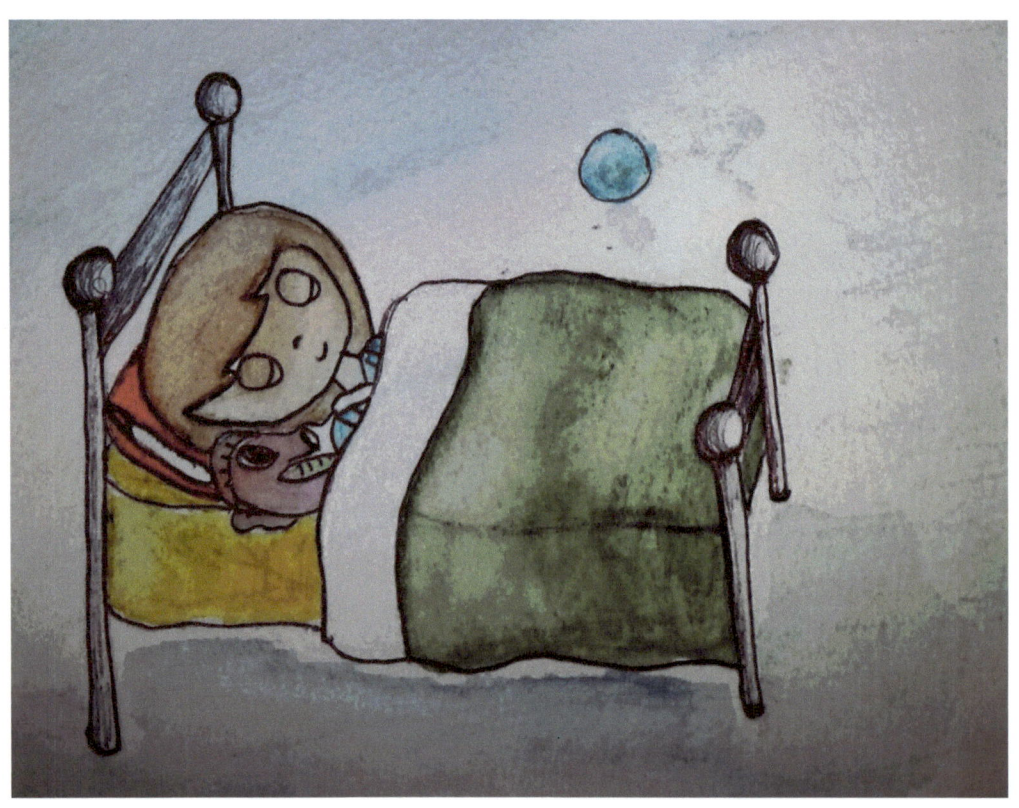

Oscar was so tired he was already asleep;
Dreaming of fish swimming in the ocean deep.
Swimming and splashing, laughing and wriggling.
Oh what fun, he couldn't stop giggling!

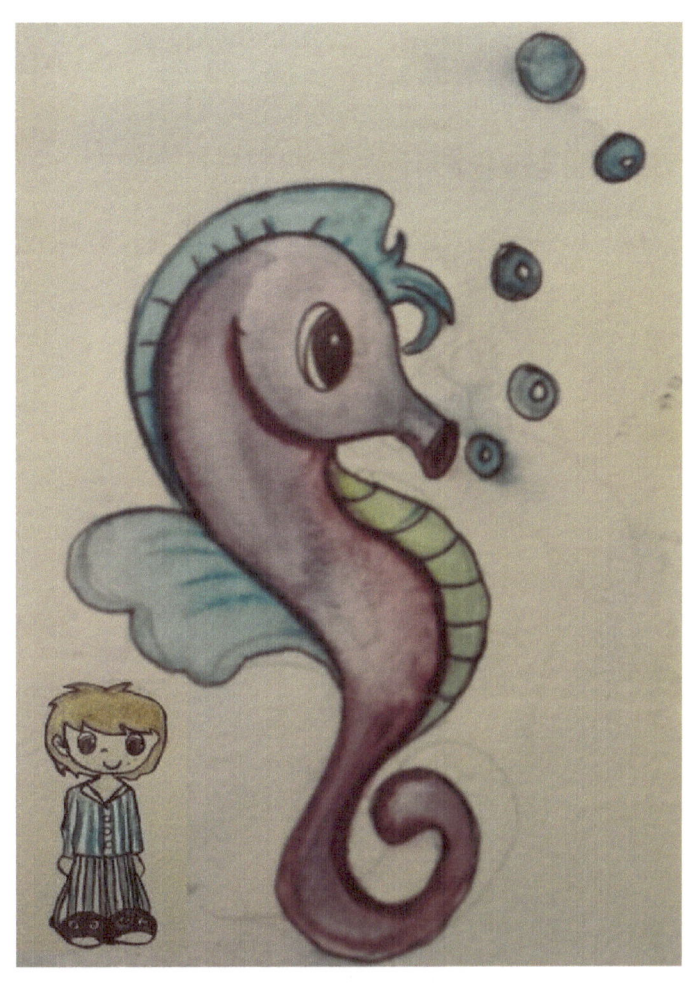

But that was until Sammy appeared
And said with a stern look to be feared:
"Oscar you haven't stretched at all tonight
You need to, or your muscles will be so tight"

Oscar looked down, shook his head in dismay,
For you see he really did not know the way
Stretching was all such a mystery to him
He would rather just play and enjoy his swim

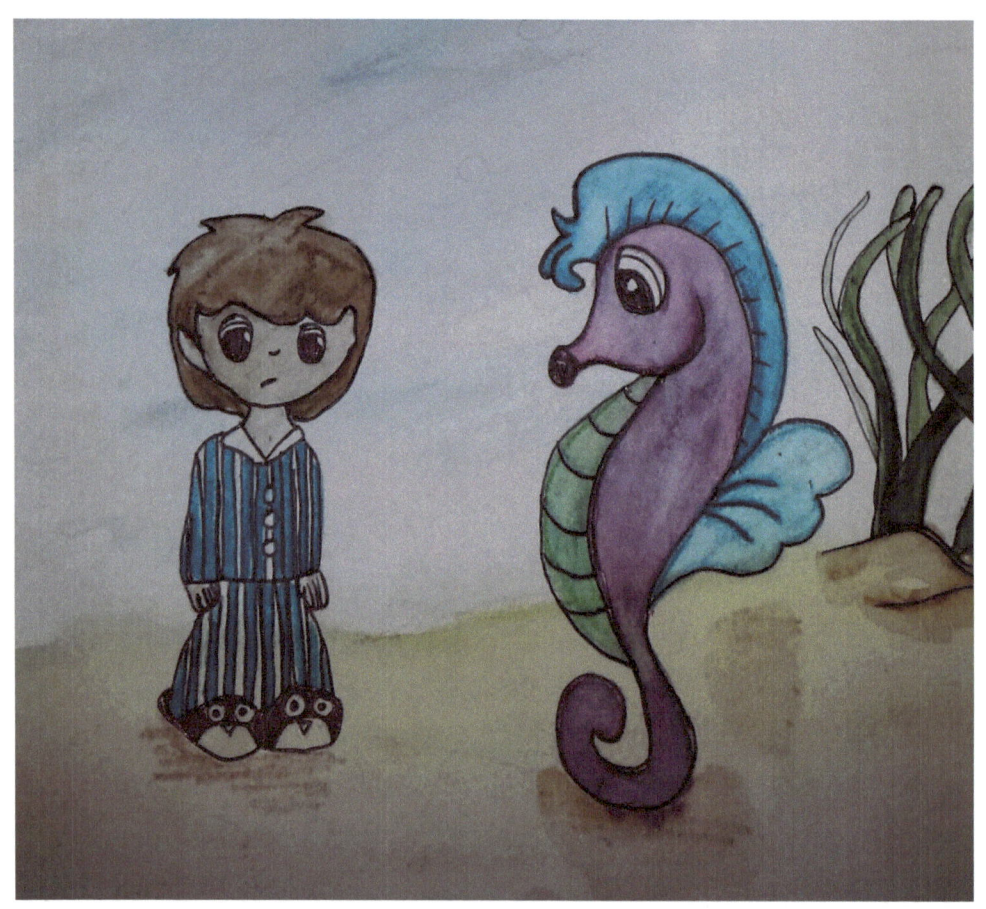

Sammy realised his friend's plight,
But deep down inside he knew he was right,
Grabbed his friend's hand and, leading the way,
Took Oscar Ocean down to a deep sea bay.

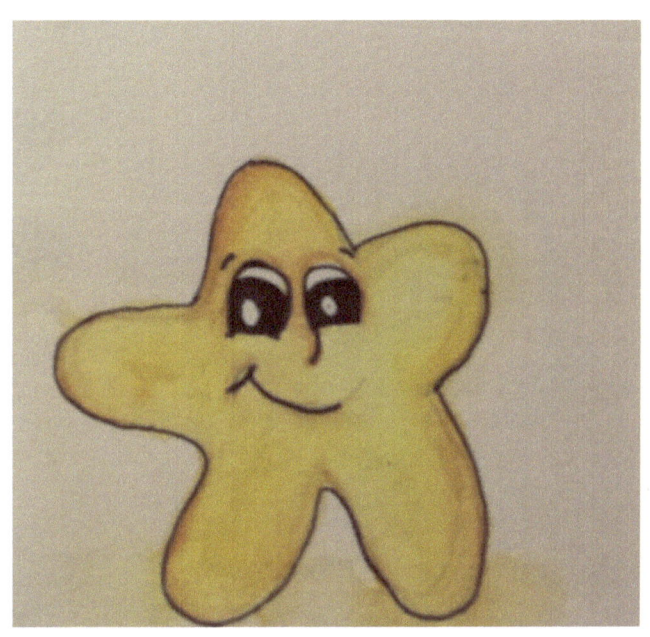

Suddenly Sidney Starfish jumped out
And cried, "Oscar my friend, why the sad
pout?"
Sammy explained the challenge ahead.
But Sidney just laughed and then kindly said:

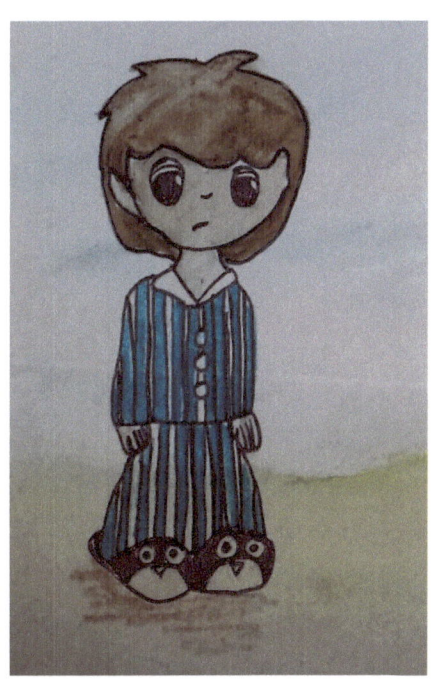

"No need to worry, we sea folks stretch all the time
Come with me Oscar and you will be fine."
Sidney Starfish was wise and finding a space
Said to Oscar, "Come on young fella, pick up the pace."

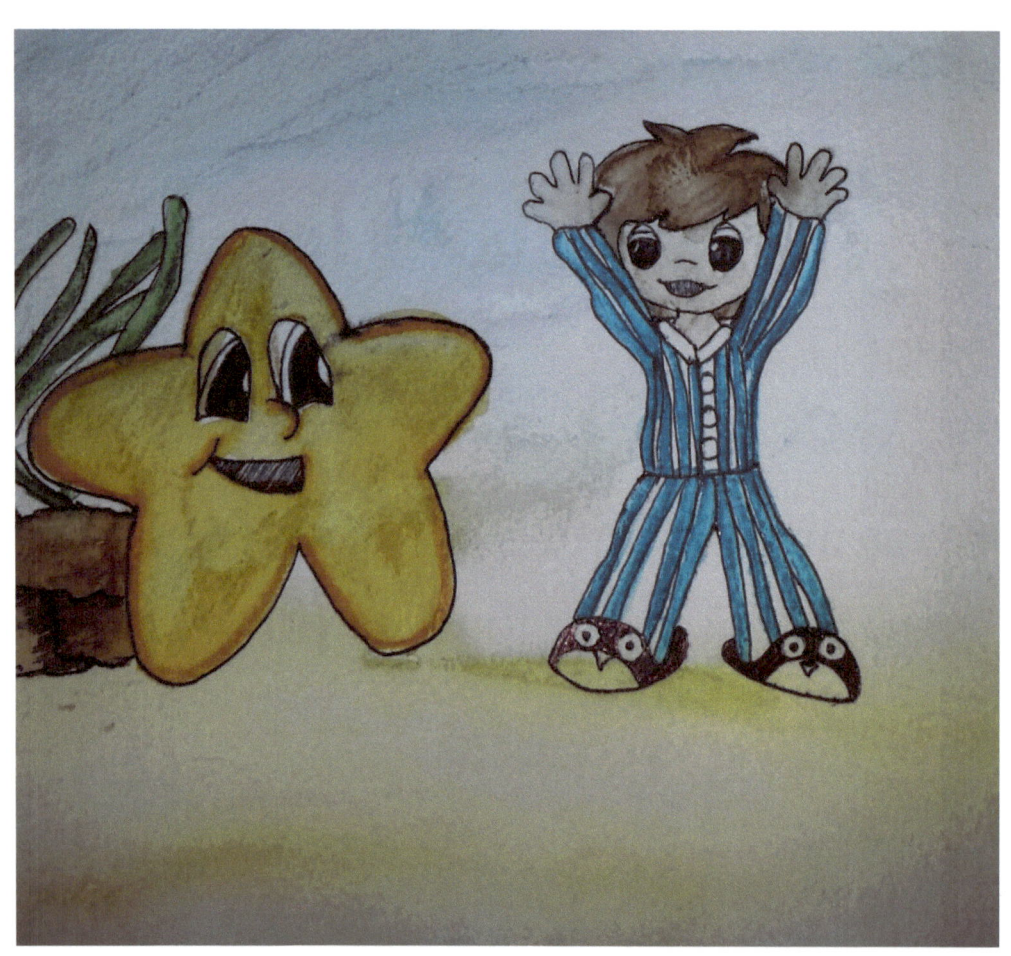

"Stretch number one is mine. You'll soon see,
Lay down and point your arms and legs out like
me
Point all those fingers, point all those toes,
Count to fifteen and there ya goes!"

Oscar felt a bit better and ready to go on
The next stretch adventure would not be long
They swam and they swam 'til they found a
sunken boat,
There they saw Olga Urchin forming a float.

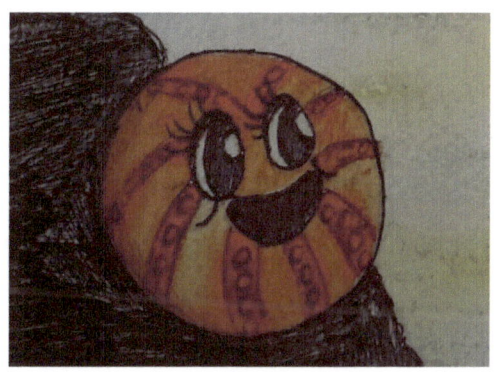

"A stretch please, Olga!" Sammy exclaimed,
"For Oscar is learning from me", he explained

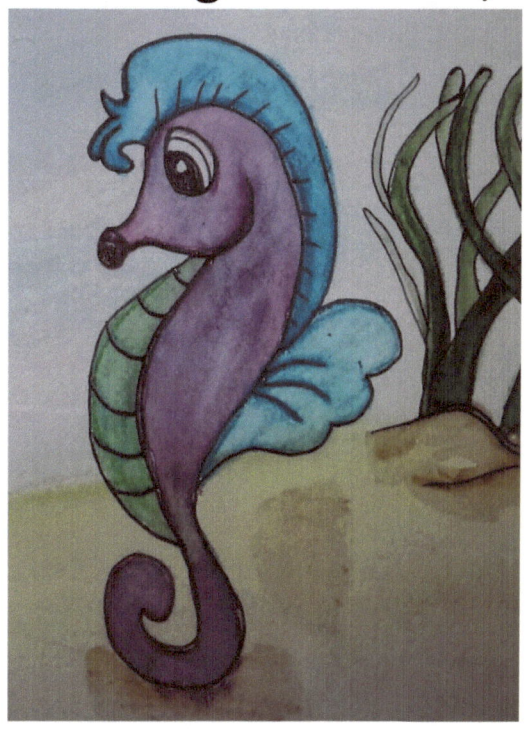

Olga smiled and lovingly said,
"Fold your arms right over your head,
Tuck in your chin, curl yourself into a ball
Now scrunch up tight legs, elbows and all.

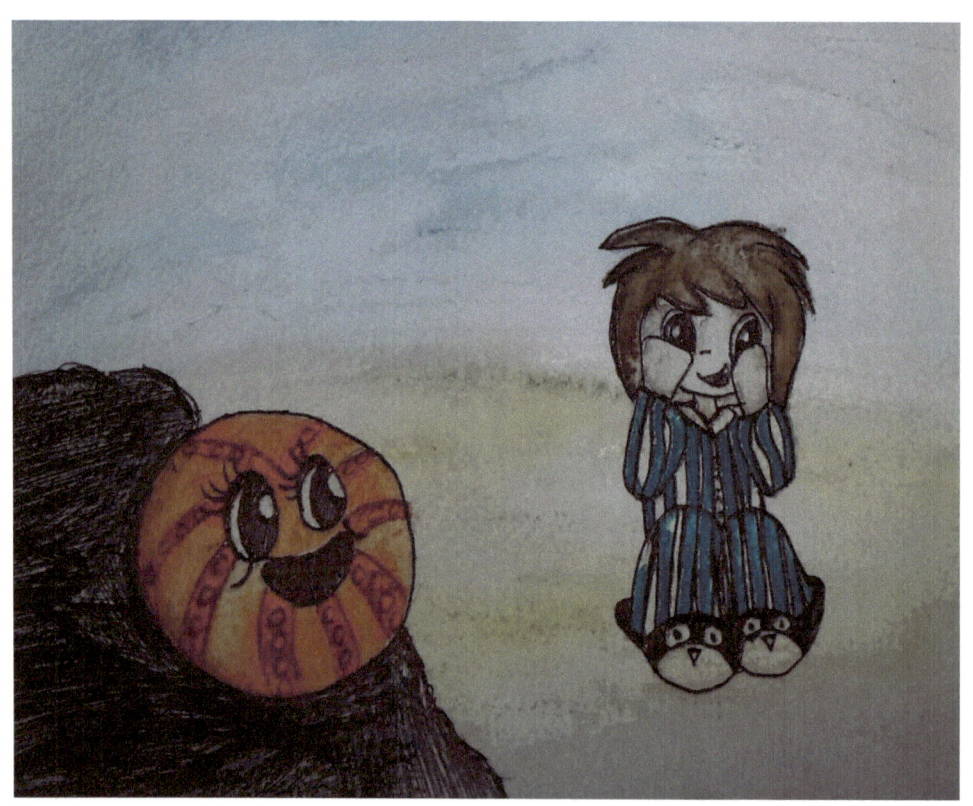

"Hold it all steady, count slowly to ten
Feel it stretch down your back muscles, and
then
Your stretch is complete!
Uncurl, then repeat."

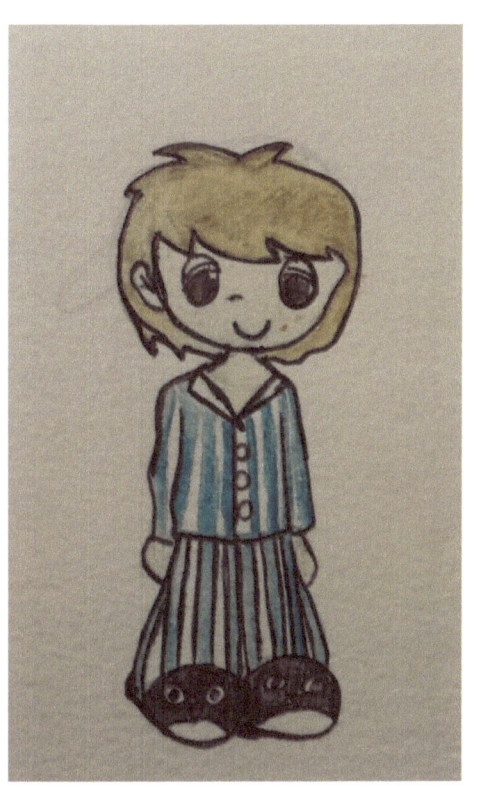

Thanking Olga, and saying goodbye,
Oscar admitted he felt energized.
Word had got round through the ocean town,
Emily Eel appeared and just lay face down.

"Copy me Oscar," Emily said,
"Lay on your belly and raise up your head.
Bring your arms straight up and lift them high
Raise your legs too as if to the sky.

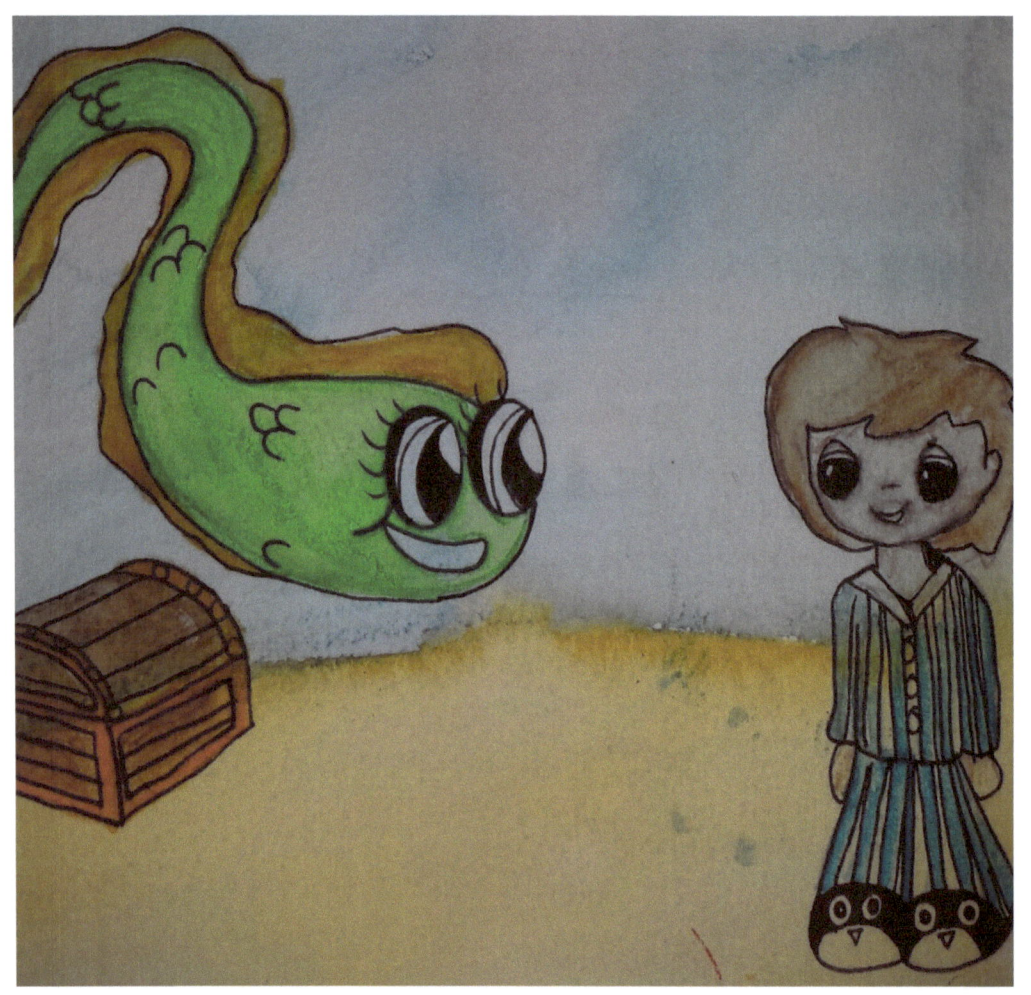

"Balancing on belly, point fingers and toes,
Breath out through our mouth and in through
the nose.
Now twist to the left and twist to the right
That's it now Oscar, you're stretching tonight!"

"Now my turn Oscar", said Sammy his friend,
"Stand on one leg and give your knee a bend,
Foot touching bottom and balancing clear,
Take one hand and hold onto your ear."

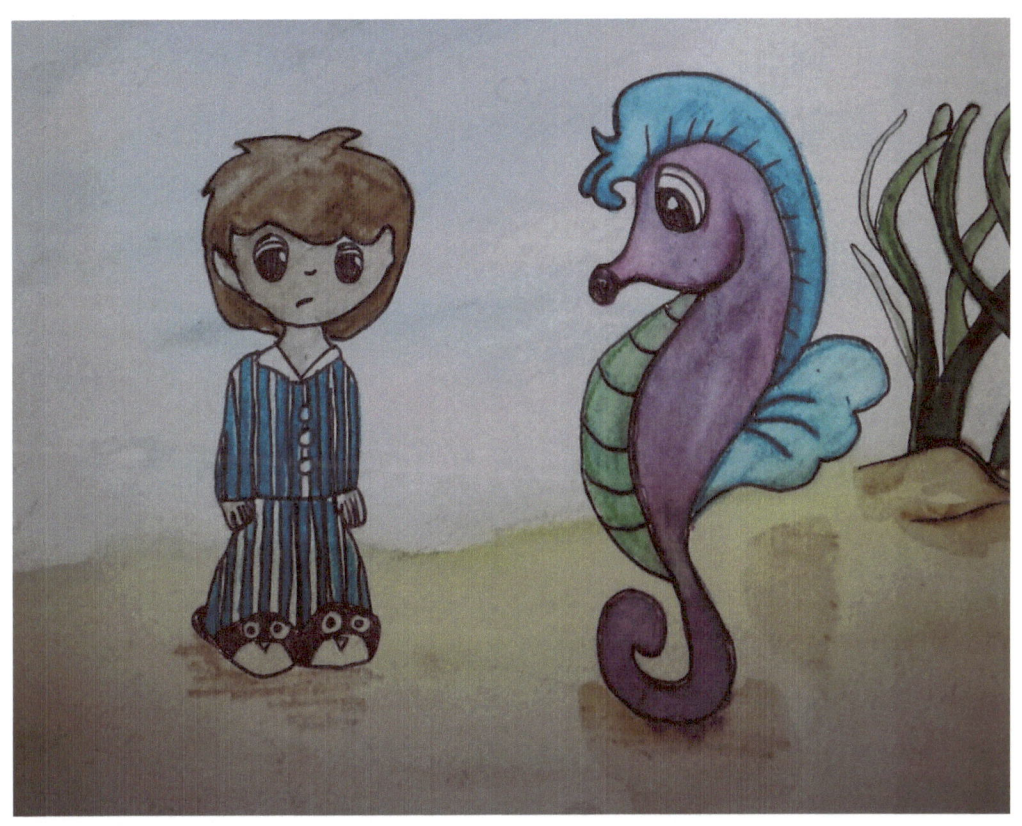

"Then swap over legs so they both have a turn,
Holding and counting, do you feel the burn?
Well now Oscar we're nearing the end,
Four stretches you've learned, my two-legged
friend."

"But one still is missing! Now let me see,
Stretch number five: Oh what could that be?"
In Jessie Jellyfish she did glide,
And calmly hovered by Oscar's side.

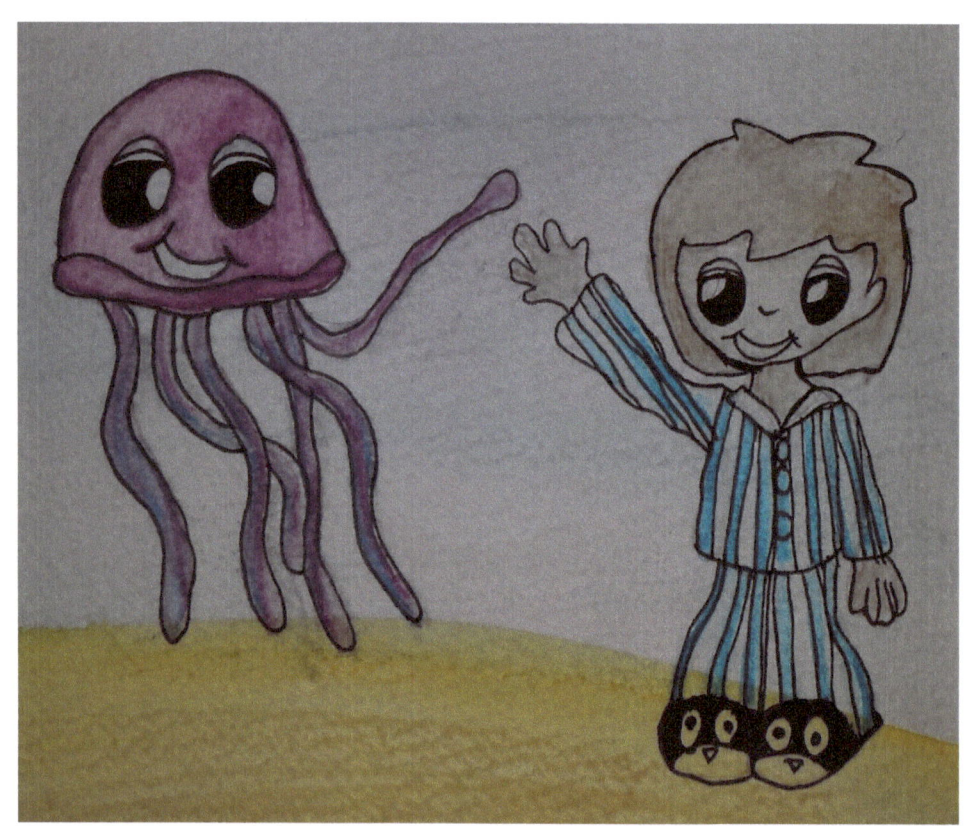

"Stretch number five is the big shake out
Wibble and wobble and shake all about.
Shake out those arms, legs and head
And then you can swim on back to your bed."

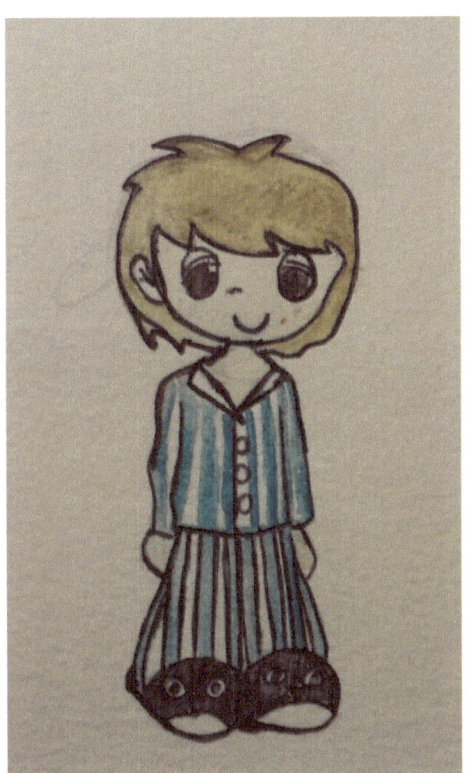

"Thank you so much all." Oscar cried,
"I feel so great now and super-energized,
And now I can see it's important for me
Stretching every day helps to keep me
healthy."

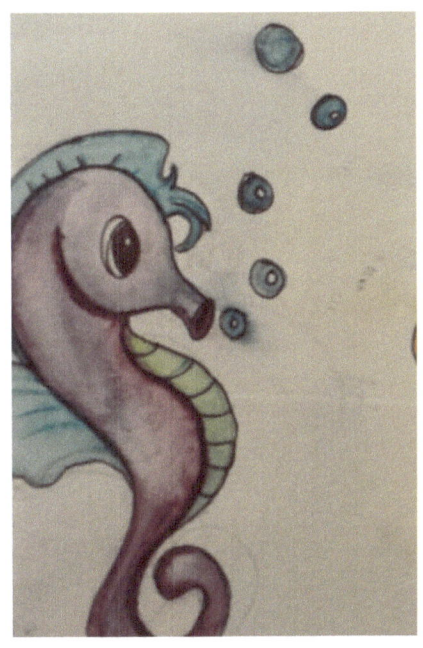

Stretching out before bed you see
Helps keep you happy, fit and healthy.
So if you want better energy,
Copy Oscar's friends from the deep blue
sea!

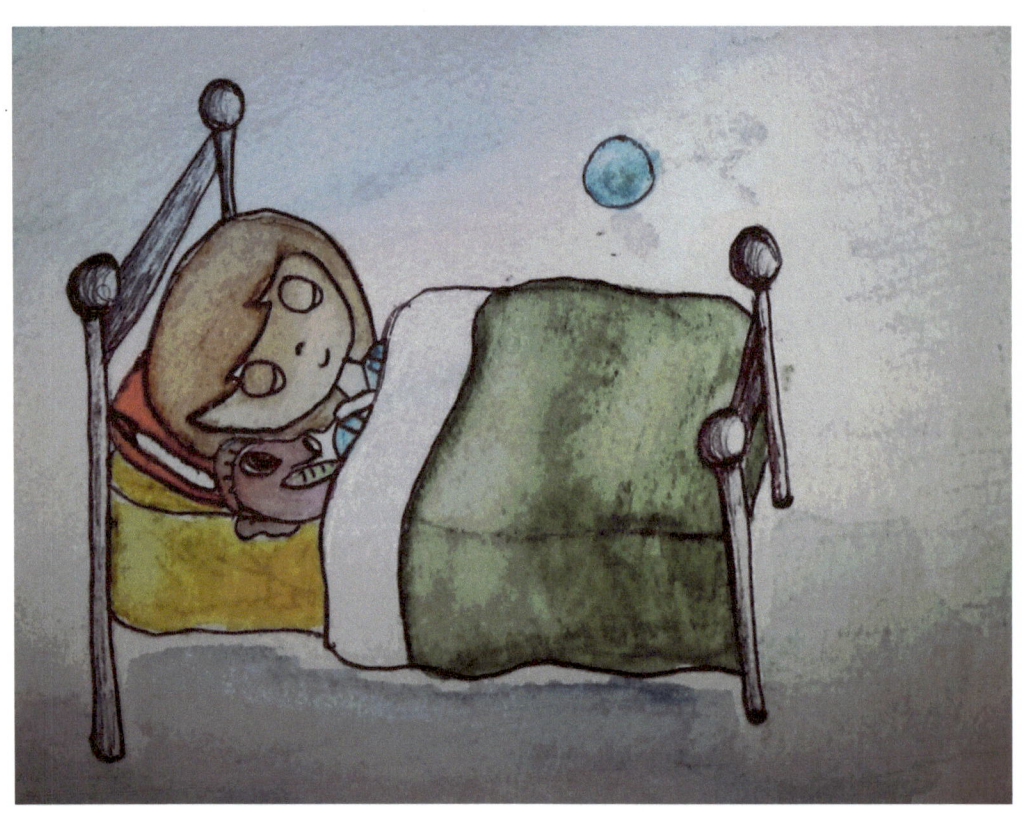

About the Author

Josephine NC Groenhart (Jo) first developed Oscar Ocean in 2010. Jo had been working at a thriving wellness centre and noticed that many parents and children didn't realise the importance of stretching or the role this has to play in leading a healthy lifestyle. She noticed on observing infants that they naturally stretch all the time, it's *in their programming*. However as we grow older we lose this good habit, through sitting more and generally moving less. As education is vital in the early years, it makes sense to encourage good lifestyle habits and to educate our children further on why it's so important.

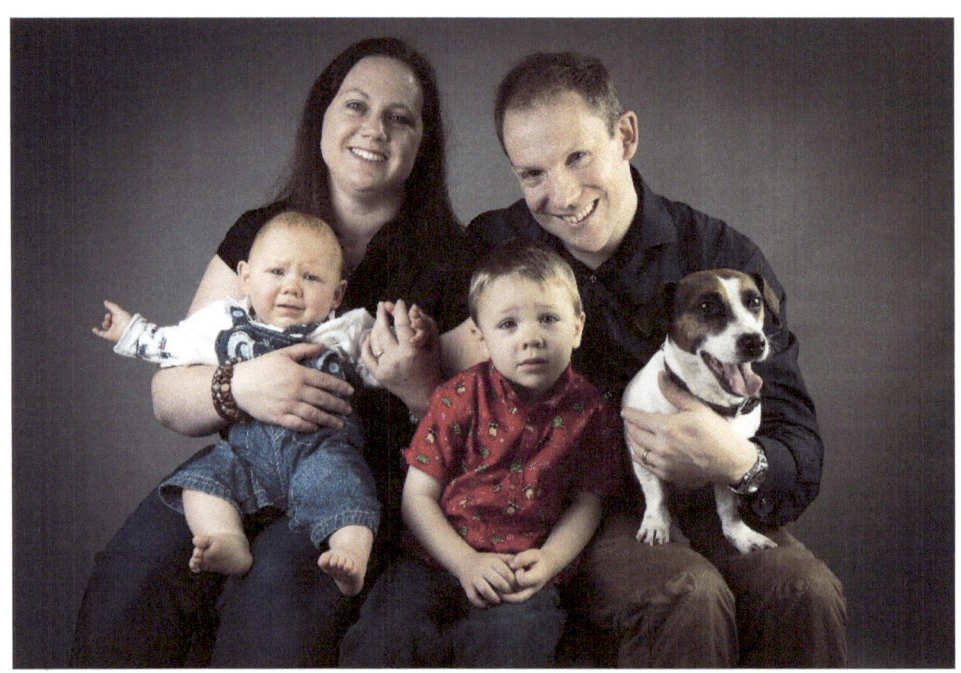

Jo currently lives in Cambridgeshire with her husband Ed, two sons, Isaac and Oakley, and dog, Izzy. Managing their busy family wellness centre and seeing her own client base has given her an opportunity to help families create their own wellness lifestyle.

Follow the progress of the rest of Oscar's journey at www.facebook.com/jo.groenhart or on twitter @JoGroenhart

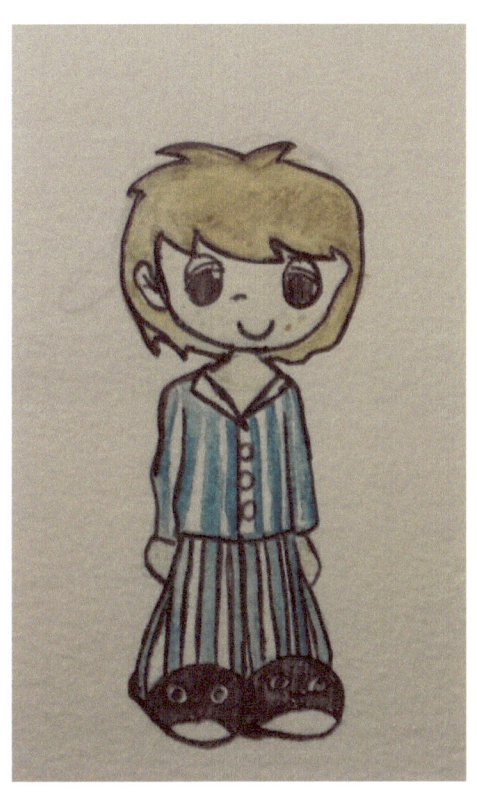

Oscar Ocean

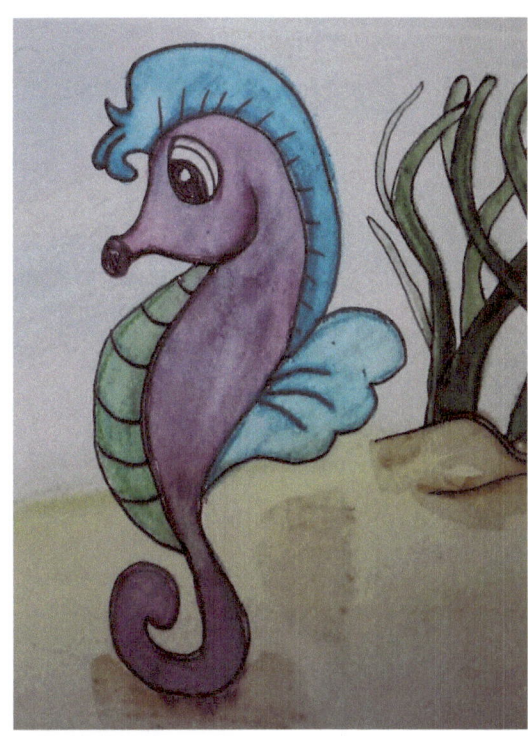

Sammy Seahorse

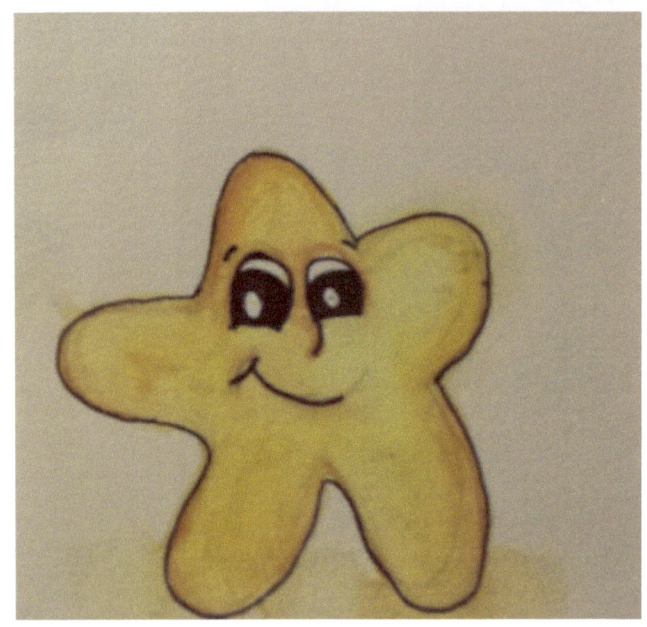

Sidney Starfish

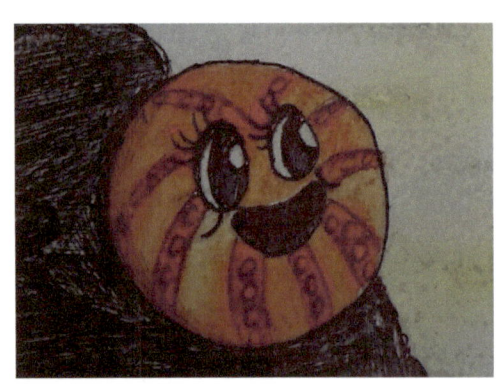

Olga Urchin

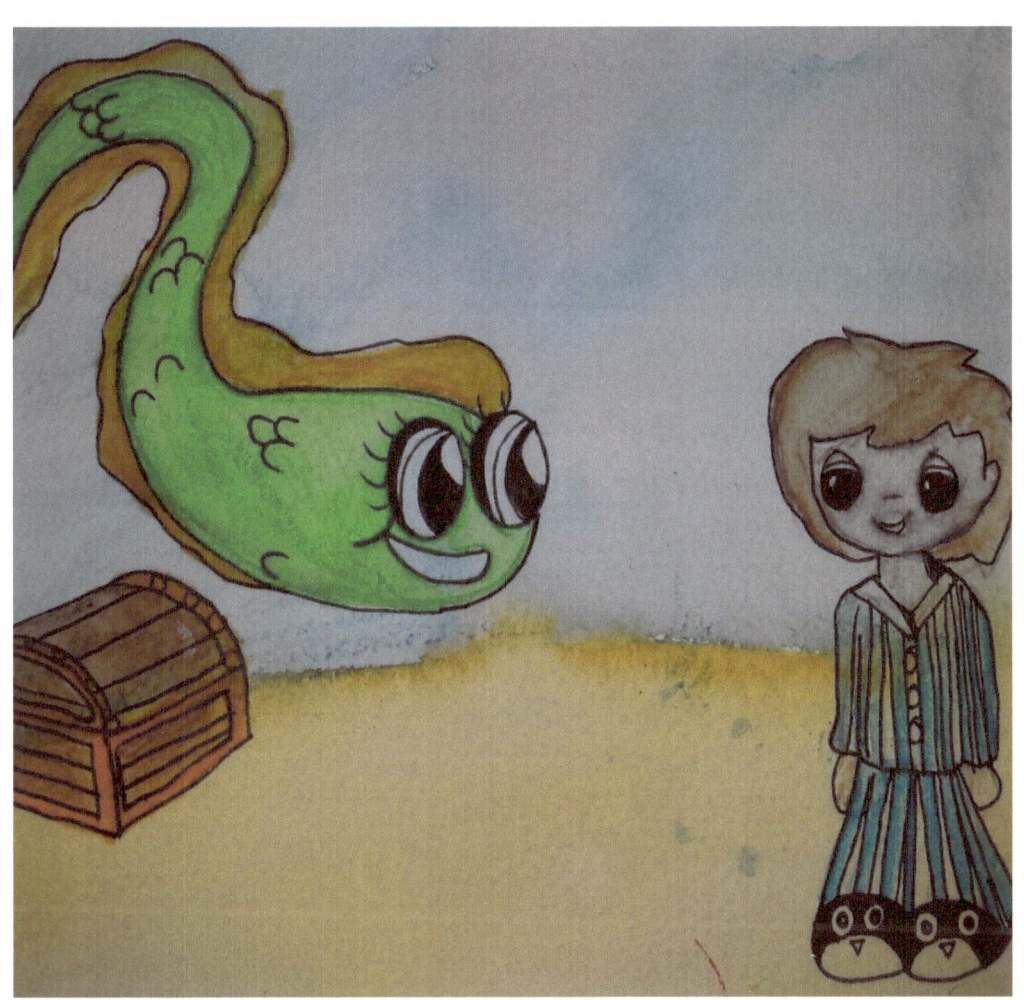

Emily Eel

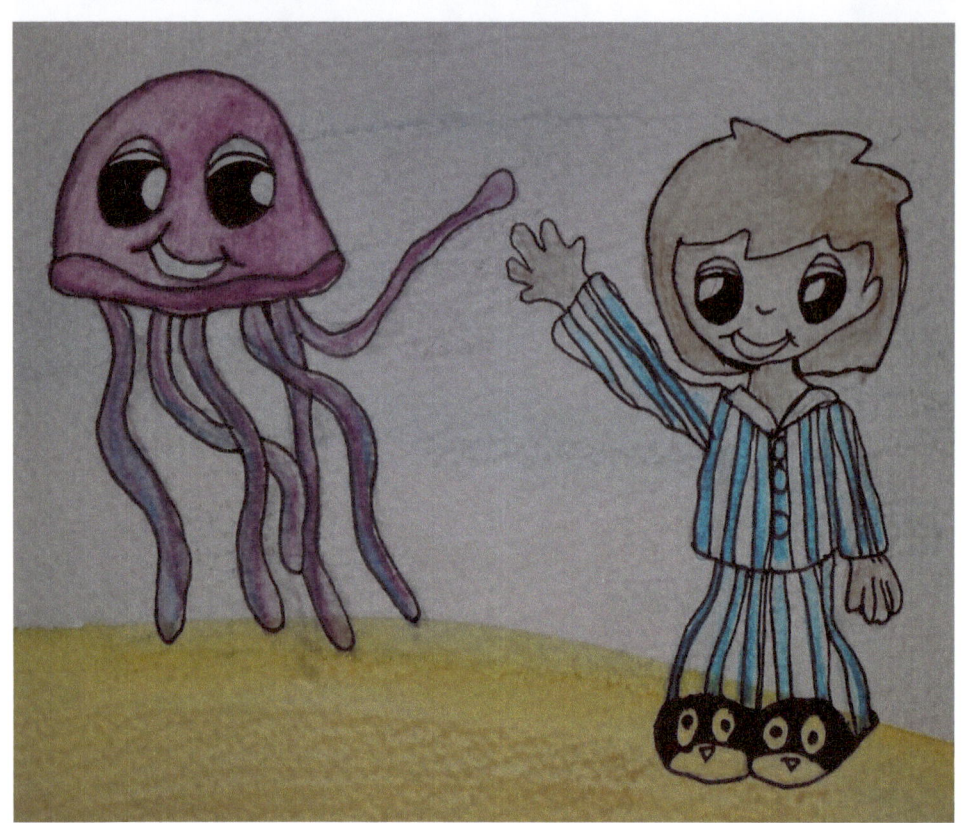

Jessie Jellyfish

Oscar Ocean and The Big Feast

Next in the Oscar Ocean and The Big Idea series, we see Oscar being taken on a journey of discovery to learn the importance of nutrition as part of a healthy lifestyle.

Available on Kindle 28th February 2015 and in print 30th March 2015.

Follow the twitter feed @JoGroenhart or Facebook page
www.facebook.com/jo.groenhart

4 Week Stretch Diary

Put a tick in the table below each day to show when you have done your stretches

Day	Stretch Complete
Monday	
Tuesday	
Wednesday	
Thursday	
Friday	
Saturday	
Sunday	

4 Week Stretch Diary

Put a tick in the table below each day to show when you have done your stretches

Day	Stretch Complete
Monday	
Tuesday	
Wednesday	
Thursday	
Friday	
Saturday	
Sunday	

4 Week Stretch Diary

Put a tick in the table below each day to show when you have done your stretches

Day	Stretch Complete
Monday	
Tuesday	
Wednesday	
Thursday	
Friday	
Saturday	
Sunday	

4 Week Stretch Diary

Put a tick in the table below each day to show when you have done your stretches

Day	Stretch Complete
Monday	
Tuesday	
Wednesday	
Thursday	
Friday	
Saturday	
Sunday	